Tea Cleanse

Shed 10 Pounds in 10 Days with the Weight Loss Miracle Plan

Table of Contents

Introduction

I want to thank you and congratulate you for downloading the book, *"Tea Cleanse: Shed 10 Pounds in 10 Days with the Weight Loss Miracle Plan."*

Can this book actually help me lose weight? Can I even lose weight by drinking tea? And can this book make weight loss as easy as it makes it sound? Yes, yes and ohh yes it will. The strategies and steps outlined in this book will show you how to improve your health tremendously with simply a cup of tea. No, not only one cup of tea silly – we haven't found that miracle potion as yet but what this book is a pretty close second. This book will provide you with everything you need to shape your body with a few instructions properly followed. Tea on its own has numerous health benefits and equipped with the right plan makes it almost impossible not to work. Obesity lately has been on the rise and a good way to counteract that is with the consumption of tea on a regular basis. Yes tea! Teas supports weight loss and also acts as a suppressant in those times of weakness. Another proven benefit that tea has is that it can boost your mood making you fill a lot more energies and healthy. The list of what tea can do for you can go on and on but i believe that you've gotten the point – tea works miracles. Read thought this book carefully and take note of the secrets that have been planted in each chapter and use your new knowledge to create the life you want.

Thanks again for downloading this book, I hope you enjoy it!

Tea Cleanse Overview

Are you looking to lose weight, improve health or you just want that extra energy to tackle your day? I know I did- I've searched and tried a variety of exercise programs and diets to hit just one of those things and I know you have too. Tea, however, is one of the best and most proven ways to not only get amazing weight loss results but also improve health considerably. Located throughout Asia tea (true tea) comes from a shrub like plant known as *Camellia Sinensis*. The leaves from this plant is what is processed to produce green, black and oolong tea which are some of the most beneficial and popular tea types in the world. The benefits that drinking tea provides, even if it's one cup a day is remarkable and almost limitless to say the least. As time goes on research is beginning to show how beneficial tea really is and we're starting to see unfold before us the range of health benefits that we can profit from. Known as the second most popular beverage in the world tea has the power to prevent cancer, promote weight loss, support dental health, boost your metabolism, lower the risk of stroke and heart disease just to name a few. Clearly, as I said previously, the benefits of drinking tea is practically limitless.

Although drinking tea provides more value to your overall health than any other beverage not all the different tea types have as many nutritional value as the next. Knowing what tea to drink to affect weight loss for example is critical. Knowing also how to brew these marvelous health miracles will be something to take note of in order to maximize their benefit which is a step that some persons tend to miss. All these and more will be explained in detail throughout the book as you learn how to increase your health and lose some pounds.

So how does it all work? Modern science has discovered nature's "healing agent" and it is known as polyphenols which tea is found to be high in. What are those you ask? For one they are antioxidants that help prevent diseases and basically keep you prone to any type of health problem. "Polyphenols protect cells and body chemicals against damage caused by free radicals—reactive atoms that contribute to tissue damage in the body. For example, when low-density lipoprotein (LDL) cholesterol is oxidized, it can become glued to arteries and cause coronary heart disease" Said Dalia Akramiene, a physiologist at Kaunas University of Medicine in Lithuania. Just to stress a little more on how beneficial this is studies have also shown that drinking tea consistently can even prevent aging. Wow right? When I found that out I thought to myself is there anything this can't do? From lowering the risk of several diseases to weight loss and now to turning back the wheel of time. Again wow!

From the past decade tea has been increasing in popularity and that it should based on what you've read so far. Although tea alone will not give you the perfect health but combined with a few healthy foods it puts you right on track to a longer, healthier and better life. Studies have shown that people who had 3-5 cups of tea daily were less prone to any type of illness/disease than those that didn't drink any type of tea.

Now let us speak on the weight loss benefits that tea provides. Yes tea is great for lowering the risk of diseases but one of the main reasons these natural cleanse agents are highly sought out after is due to its fat burning and weight reducing properties. The vitamins and antioxidants that tea contains have the ability to speed up your metabolism, making it easier to burn fat throughout the day. It also gets rid of the toxins in the body that hinder the fat burning process which definitely increases the rate of weight loss but not only that tea enhances brain functions which increases your alertness, focus and keeps you energized. This will make it easier to stick to diets and have you more capable and effective during workouts. Tea also includes caffeine (not as much as your typical Monday morning coffee) but this will help the metabolic rate so you can lose weight faster when exercising. So what can you expect while on a tea cleanse diet? The first point is a very obvious one- you must drink quite a few cups of tea on a daily basis. The more tea you drink the better for you. Second you must still acknowledge the fact that this isn't a magic potion that will do it all for you with hardly any effort from you. Although it is the simplest way

I've seen weight loss done, I would like to inform you that anything worth doing is worth doing it well so be prepared for changes; both in your diet and results. Also depends on what your current diet is like you may feel a bit tired and irritable in the first few days of this cleanse but that's all normal. This is telling you that the toxins are leaving your body and cleaning out your system. Bare patience for the first couple of days and by the fourth day you will begin to feel more energized as your body gets accustom to the change. Trust me when I say it's worth it.

Natural Teas- All you need to Know

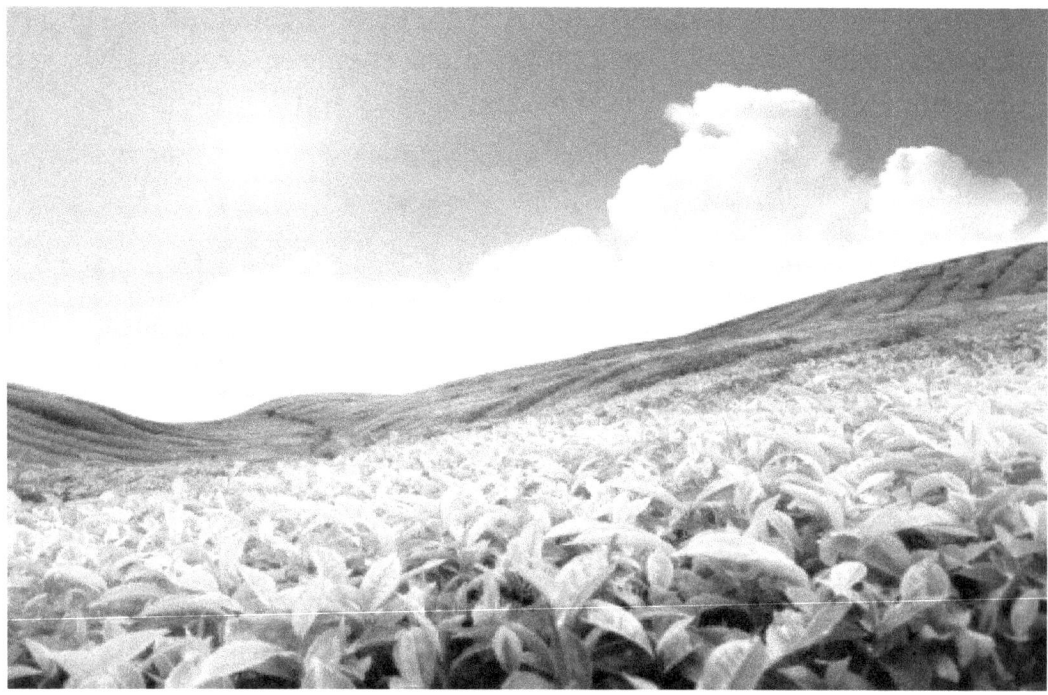

In the first chapter as much as we spoke about the benefits of tea and other information pertaining to how it does what is does there was very little said on the different tea types. So what is tea exactly? Some of this may have already been covered in the first chapter but you might have been fully aware. Real tea comes from a single plant- the *Camellia Sinensis* which is used to create the different types of tea. Many people mistake certain herbs for tea and are often confused by their similarities for instance the herb Rooibos also know as red tea is frequently mistaken for a tea but is not a true tea. The difference between the two is that herbs come from a variety of plants whereas tea is only made from one plant and can be classified under the headings of green tea, white tea, yellow tea, black tea, oolong tea and pu'erh tea. Although they are all derived from one plant it's the way they are processed which makes them different. Most herbs also have no caffeine. Despite this book is called tea cleanse some herbs will be included such as the Rooibos herb which we will talk more about later in this chapter.

What's best for Weight Loss and Health?

As I mentioned before there are a variety of teas but what tea should be used for best results? Knowing what tea is used to boost your metabolism, prevent weight gain and even prevent cravings is only the first part of achieving your weight loss goals. The second step is in the form of knowing how to prepare these miracle workers by maximizing their health benefits. So let's get started by first understanding the different tea types and what they can do for you.

Oolong tea: if you want a tea that is delicious, filled with vitamins, minerals and antioxidants that is able to promote weight loss then the oolong tea is a great choice. This nutrition packed tea is very effective at controlling the metabolism of fat in the body due to the polyphenols compounds that it has. Polyphenols are powerful antioxidants that neutralize and remove free radicals in your body which can cause serious harm to your health. Including a cup of oolong tea in your diet will make you less vulnerable to aliments that include stroke, cancer, and diabetes. Oolong tea, according to a scientific study that was done improved the skin condition of patients suffering from eczema by only drinking three cups of tea a day. This can be seen that oolong tea has beneficial substances that can improve skin care. While oolong tea has a variety of health benefits and is a great way to burn fat it tends to be high in caffeine so that's something you should take note of while monitoring your cleanse period. Caffeine works differently on people so be sure to keep that in mind if you are aware of the side-effects that caffeine has on your body but altogether oolong tea is the one to use to help burn fat.

Green tea: when it comes to weight loss green tea has replaced many western beverages because of its weight loss properties- an antioxidant known as EGCG which is helpful in treating a variety of diseases while still being able to burn fat. One of the main features that make this tea known worldwide especially in the weight loss industry is its ability to enhance the rate of metabolism, thereby encouraging a faster consumption of the fat storage of the body. And if you're serious about weight loss and have a workout routine try a cup of green tea before you start. You may just recognize a higher energy level during your sets since green tea aids in boosting stamina and endurance. So for a higher metabolism green tea is the way to go.

Peppermint tea: technically speaking peppermint is an herb and not a tea but it contains just as much benefits as any other tea types. For a relaxing evening this tasty and refreshing tea is perfect to lighten up and just kick your feet up from a hard day's work. Unlike the previous teas mentioned (green tea and oolong tea) peppermint tea is caffeine free making it a wonderful delight at the end of the day. "When it comes to stress and anxiety, peppermint tea is one of your best allies. The menthol that is naturally present in the tea is a muscle relaxant; the relaxation of the muscles can be an enormous component of natural stress and anxiety relief... not to mention falling asleep!" said an article published by the Sleuth Journal. Another thing which this tea is famous for is its power to improve digestion, eliminate inflammation, reduce pain, relax the body and mind, prevent/treat bad breath, aids in weight loss and boosts the immune system. How exactly does peppermint aids in weight loss you ask? Let me explain- in a study in the *Journal of Neurological and Orthopaedic Medicine and surgery* researchers found out that peppermint helped people lose weight simply by sniffing its scent whenever they felt hungry. The scent of peppermint acts as a suppressant to your appetite, making you feel fuller resulting in weight loss. How easy does that sound? You can literally sniff your way to a slimmer you.

White tea: if you have had conversations with people about tea or have read about tea before you may have heard some recommend green tea over white tea but it doesn't have anything to do with it being any less benefitting than green tea. Green tea is simply easier and cheaper to buy. Now that I've gotten that out of the way let me go into the details of white tea. This tea comprises of a smoother, gentler and even a slight sweet taste compared to green tea and is a major health enhancer. This tea is the least processed amongst the varying tea types and it's because of this white tea carries more antioxidants. Health benefits of white tea consist of reduced risk of cancer, cardiovascular disorder, improvement in oral health and also it has anti-aging properties which help in maintaining healthy, youthful skin. For people with little time to exercise but want to lose weight including a few cups of white tea in your diet will prove to work wonders. Studies suggest that white tea provides evidence of a possible anti-obesity effect. During several experiments the tea showed prevention of adipogenesis which is the process where fat cells are formed. So if you want to drop a few pounds with white tea's ability to inhibit the generation of fat you will be on your way to success. When brewing white tea it is best done with the actual loose leaves rather than tea bags. This guarantees the presents of more nutrients and therefore health benefits. Since tea bags have undergone more processing the process may have extracted some of the nutrients and antioxidants it contains.

Pu-erh tea: this tea is one which has been in the Chinese culture for a very long time due to it being a tremendous health enhancer especially with weight loss. Pu-erh tea is a great weight loss tea and has stood its grounds with the other well known teas throughout the years because of its ability to metabolize fat and help shed pounds. Although this tea is great for weight loss if it is consumed at the wrong times it can have the opposite effect on your body hence the reason you should pay close attention to the instructions when preparing and consuming pu-erh tea. I will speak more in detail of how this tea should be brewed for maximized effect later in this book but knowing the times pu-erh teas should be drunk is critical. It is said that a cup of pu-erh tea is most effective at reducing weight when taken an hour after meals. The properties of pu-erh tea are able to remove excess grease and help your body eliminate surplus hard-to-digest fats. If taken just before meals the tea will have an opposite effect on your body. The fat deposits that are in your body and any residue found in your stomach will be cleared up if taken an hour before meals. But wait, if it clears out the fat in your system how is that a bad thing? For one this effect will most definitely increase your appetite and cause you to eat more (unless you have a strong willpower). So sticking to this tea after meals is what will bring results. Another important point with this tea is that when you begin drinking it the tea might bring about sudden hunger pangs which I recommend should be eased with fresh fruits, salads or just plain vegetables. After a period of time your stomach will adapt to your new diet and the hunger pangs will go away. All in all pu-erh tea is great to speed up digestion and remove fat before it can be absorbed by the body.

Rooibos tea: located in South Africa also known as "red tea" rooibos comes from the leaves of the *spalathus linearis* bush plant. This tea is red in color as you may have guessed already and is extremely low in calories- 2 calories to be precise when there's no extra added sugar. And if you're worried about the taste especially after not adding sugar- don't be because this beverage is naturally sweet making it a delight for easy weight loss. Just as the other teas mention rooibos tea has an abundance of health benefits varying from cures for nagging headaches, insomnia, asthma, eczema, bone weakness, hypertension, allergies, and premature aging. How can this tea be any better? I'll tell you how- it's caffeine free for those who have a hard time staying asleep at night. We all know that sleep is an important aspect in our weight loss goals. Not only because lack of sleep affects how energized we are throughout the day but also because it affects hunger and fullness hormones which may cause problems with weight loss. What's more, rooibos tea contains a compound called aspalathin which research shows can reduce stress hormones that cause hunger and fat storage and are linked to other illnesses such as hypertension, metabolic syndrome, cardiovascular disease, insulin resistance and type 2 diabetes. A delicious tea that regulates fat-hormones is just what you need in your diet. On average a typical American drinks approximately 3 cups of coffee per day. If one of those cups is substituted with a cup of rooibos tea you would lose about 7.5 pounds per annum and that's just adding only one cup a day. How great would the results be if you drunk even more a day?

Hibiscus tea: I'm sure that you have heard of hibiscus tea before. I mean who hasn't with its ruby red color and its vast range of health benefits? Hibiscus tea relieves from high blood pressure, high cholesterol, as well as inflammatory problems. But this tea does not stop there as it also has anti-cancer properties and anti-depressant properties. Carrying no caffeine and very little calories hibiscus tea is also very well recognized as a natural diuretic. We all know that water is important in any diet but too much water in your diet can also have you feeling uncomfortable and this tea's diuretic properties is able to rid your body of excess water and prevent temporary bloating. So what's the link between hibiscus tea and weight loss? The production of amylase is inhibited by compounds contained in hibiscus tea. What this means is that it prevents the absorption of starch and glucose in the body that causes you to gain weight. Lowering the amount of amylase in the body is a sure way to shed some pounds. It's no wonder hibiscus is found in many weight loss products. As beneficial as this tea is there are a few points that you should take note of such as hibiscus tea is not recommended by women who are pregnant. It has been said that this tea due to emmenagogue effects may stimulate menstruation or blood flow in the uterus. Another side effect with some people is the feeling of being intoxicated so it's recommended that you know how the tea affects you before doing any driving or dangerous activity. After you know how this tea affects your body and all signs are good enjoying a few cups of this cranberry flavored drink is a great way to lose weight while the pounds just slide off.

Black tea: known for its medicinal qualities black tea is one of the most common teas known to man. Black tea is a pure tea and what differentiates in from green tea or white tea is in the way it is processed. When being processed black tea is fermented and oxidized which gives it its unique flavor and color. Jam-packed with antioxidants, minerals, vitamins and other important nutrients black tea is capable of positively impacting high cholesterol, diarrhea, tooth decay, low-concentration levels, digestive problems, poor blood circulation, high blood pressure, and asthma. When consumed in moderate amounts on a regular basis black tea also helps you relax and concentrate better. How does that sound after a long day? Black tea, since it's not as heavily caffeinated as other beverages is found to have just enough caffeine to help enhance blood flow without over stimulating the heart. Your metabolism and respiratory system may also be stimulated as well giving you an energy increase that can be useful during workouts.

Ginseng tea: ginseng has been used for centuries in Chinese medicine for stamina and increased energy levels and overall well being. There are three types of ginseng which include American, Asian and Siberian ginseng all of which are very beneficial to human health and vitality. Ginseng tea has been found to be beneficial in helping with diabetes, cancer, anxiety, cholesterol, male sexual functions, immune system support, mental performance, weight loss control and is considered to be a great health stimulant. That's quite a reputation ginseng has judging by what's mentioned so far and I'm pretty sure I left out a few other benefits of this amazing herb. Despite of its varying benefits excessive use of ginseng may cause hypertension and insomnia even though it is a nontoxic herb. Drinking ginseng continuously and consistently for periods longer than 90 days is not recommended. When used for several weeks it is advised to go at least a week without it. Taking ginseng for weight loss however has become a popular practice as it is a natural appetite suppressant helping you lose and control your weight. It is also good for people looking to boost their metabolic rate to shed a few pounds and burn fat at a high rate.

Rose tea: roses are usually known for their beauty and sweet aroma but they are equally matched with what's on the inside as well. These decorative pieces are filled with natural antioxidants, minerals and vitamins such as vitamin E that is beneficial for healthy skin. Rose tea is also great for constipation and diarrhea, stress, digestion, developing a strong immune system and fights infections. Rose tea with fruit flavors such as lemon and orange is a healthy way to keep your sugar cravings at bay and prevent you from adding any actual sugar in your diet which we all know further aids in weight loss.

Summary (what does what)

In this summary I will be briefly going over what tea is best used for what purpose. Each tea mentioned in this chapter has a variety of health benefits but as you may be aware of some have a greater effect in certain areas than others and just in case it wasn't clear to you before this will give you a chance to recognize the each tea's most beneficial function.

Metabolism Boosting Teas

As the name suggest these teas have been found to be the best at boosting your metabolism rate for you to be burning calories like crazy.

- Green tea
- Oolong tea
- Pu-erh tea
- Black tea
- Ginseng tea

Stress Relieving Teas

One of the wonderful things about teas is its ability to ease your days and take away your worries by placing you in a calm and relaxed state. Stress relieving teas make it easy to sleep well at night and wake up feeling wonderful and at peace.

- Peppermint tea
- Rooibos tea
- Hibiscus tea
- Black tea

Appetite Suppressing Teas

What's one of the main reasons people can't achieve their health and weight loss goals? Cravings- this is what majority of people suffer from and teas that contain properties to suppress your appetite is one of the best solutions. These teas crush your cravings and make it easier to lose weight.

- Peppermint tea

- Ginseng tea

Weight Reducing Teas

Generally speaking all the teas mentioned in this chapter are weight reducing but these teas are specific to reduce bloating, inflammation and constipation which allows you to lose belly fat and make weight loss seem simple as 1, 2, 3.

- White tea
- Rooibos tea
- Rose tea
- Hibiscus tea

Brewing Perfect Tea – Maximizing Weight Loss

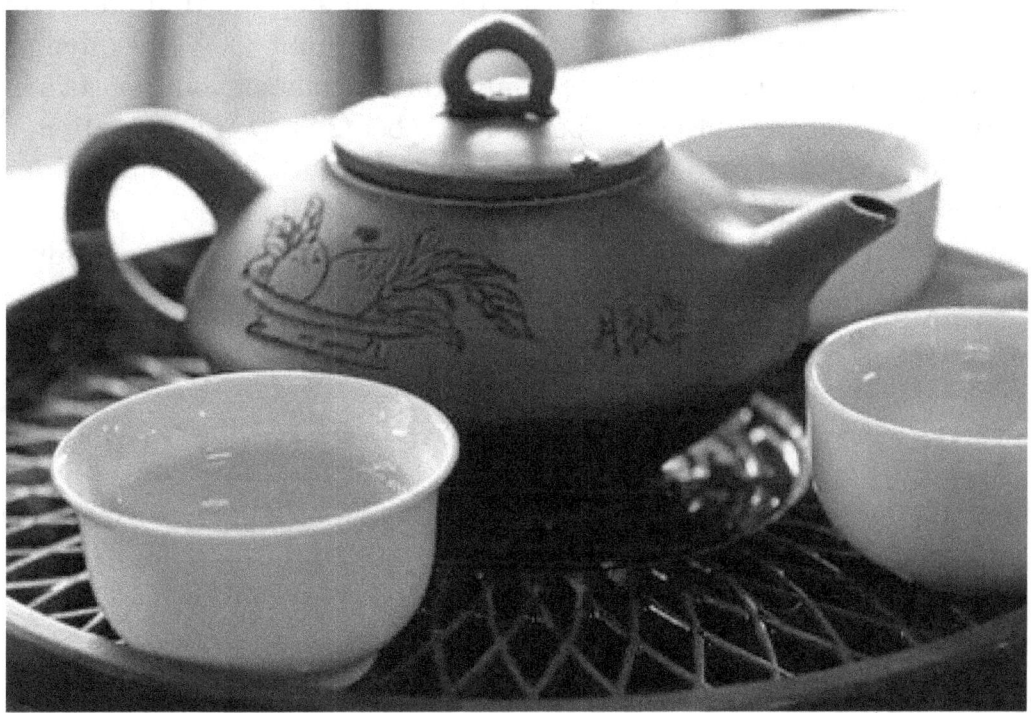

If you were asked to brew tea then I'm pretty sure you would be able to handle something like that but would you do it the best way for maximized benefits? In most Asian cultures brewing tea is an art and there are two basic methods of brewing tea. The first is known as western brewing which is what Americans are use to and the second is known as Gong Fu brewing which is a method of brewing that has been used for centuries in Chinese culture. What's the difference in the two? It's simply a matter of portion and time. Using the western technique the less tea/herb is used in brewing tea and this means that the tea has to be steeped for a longer period of time whereas in the Gong Fu way of brewing more tea/herbs are used for a lot less time.

Tea steeping is a very important process when making tea because when done right this is what will give your tea the richness in nutrients, flavor and aroma. No one likes bitter tea so let us all skip the trial and error process and get right into making perfect tea on our very first attempt. There are many factors which determine the outcome of your tea such as the tea's quality, quantity, temperature it's being brewed at, duration of infusion, the water used and even the material of the teapot. Later during the chapter I will be listing some major tips that will provide more value to your tea brewing but for now let us look at what is needed to produce quality tea.

Materials/Equipments needed to Brew Tea

Having the right set of equipments is where this brewing process begins and they are as followed:

- Teapot
- Strainer
- Thermometer
- Weight
- Cup/Pot
- Tablespoons

Specifics for Brewing Tea

The two tables will be listing the specific details for brewing tea in the two methods we spoke about earlier.

Gong Fu Brewing (150ml of water)

Type of Tea	Amount	Temperature	Time of 1st Infusion	2nd Infusion
Oolong Tea				
strip	5g	95*c	10 seconds	+5
ball	8g	95*c	20 seconds	+5
Green Tea	5g	80*c	5 seconds	+5
White Tea	5g	85*c	5 seconds	+5
Black Tea				
Small Leaf	5g	85*c	5 seconds	+5
Large Leaf	6g	95*c	10 seconds	+5
Pu-erh Tea				
Small Leaf	5g	95*c	5 seconds	+10
Large Leaf	5g	95*c	5 seconds	+10
Herbal Tea	5g	95*c	5 seconds	+10

Maximum number of infusions

5 times- white tea, green tea

6 times- oolong tea (strip)

8 times- oolong tea (ball), black tea (small and large leaf)

20 times- pu-erh tea (small and large leaf), herbal tea

Western Brewing (300ml of water)

Type of Tea	Amount	Temperature	Time of 1st Infusion	2nd Infusion
Oolong Tea				
strip	2g	95*c	90 seconds	+30
ball	3.5g	95*c	120 seconds	+30
Green Tea	2g	80*c	120 seconds	+60
White Tea	2g	85*c	180 seconds	+60
Black Tea				
Small Leaf	2.5g	95*c	90 seconds	+60
Large Leaf	2.5g	95*c	90 seconds	+60
Pu-erh Tea				
Small Leaf	2.5g	95*c	120 seconds	+30
Large Leaf	2.5g	95*c	120 seconds	+30
Herbal Tea	2.5g	95*c	120 seconds	+30

Maximum number of infusions

2 times- white tea,

3 times- green tea

4 times- black tea (small and large leaf), oolong tea (strip)

5 times- oolong tea (ball)

6 times- pu-erh tea (small and large leaf), herbal tea

Steps Involve in Brewing

STEP 1: fill your kettle up with fresh water and heat it to the appropriate temperature for the tea you're brewing. Use a thermometer to measure the required temperature.

STEP 2: preheat the teapot you're going to steep the tea in by swirling a little of the hot water in and then dispose of the water after you believe the teapot is properly preheated. Doing this will keep the teapot at the temperature needed to steep the tea. The temperature might decrease if the teapot is not preheated and affect the infusion process of the tea.

STEP 3: rinse the tea leaves with the water as well. This softens the tea leaves and makes it less bitter. This is recommended for darker teas.

STEP 4: place your tea leaves in the filter/strainer. Modern teapots usually have a built-in strainer but for more traditional teapots a filter should be equipped to fit perfectly into the teapot to place the tea leaves.

STEP 5: pour the right amount of water into the tea pot and cover it with the top to start the steeping process. Let it steep for the required time.

STEP 6: remove the filter with the leaves.

STEP 7: pour into your cup and let it settle to your required temperature.

STEP 8: ENJOY!

Tea Brewing Tips

- Use loose leaves- for a richer, flavorful tea it is recommended to use loose tea leaves rather than tea bags. You may find it inconvenient at first but I can assure you that is not the case. Loose leaves prepare better quality tea for maximized benefits.
- Get more with the Gong Fu method- this way of brewing used more tea/herbs to steep in less time which will make it quick and

easy to enjoy a cup of tea. This method is also considered more economical because the teas can be reused for a longer period of time giving you more for less.

- Herbal secrets- unlike real tea herbal tea doesn't get that bitter taste when it steeps for longer than suggested due to the lack of tannins in it. The longer you steep herbal teas the richer they are in antioxidants and more health enhancing nutrients.

- Do not over steep- one of the problems with brewing tea is that it is sometimes over steeped and the required times/temperatures are not followed. Please adhere to the instructions and details when brewing tea for a better result.

- Always use fresh water- fresh drawn, cold water is best when preparing tea. The water must be free from any pollutants and any other substance that may alter the taste of the tea hence the reason distilled water should never be used. Pre-heated water also falls under the "no no" category as it is most times overheated and stripped of its oxygen content which is essential for the best tasting tea.

- No microwaving tea- Microwaving the water that is used to make the tea is also a practice you will want to avoid as this is something that prevents your tea from tasting best.

- Add a little extra- If you want to add a little extra something to your tea here's a few condiments that can work wonders for black and herbal tea; black (milk, honey, sugar, lemon), herbal (honey, lemon).

- Some teas are best plain- it's always recommended that certain teas be drunk plain such as oolong tea, green tea and white tea but between you and me a little experimenting of your own won't hurt.

- Provide enough space for infusion- tea needs enough space to unfurl and make contact with the water so choosing a spacious infuser will be better for steeping allowing the leaves to swim freely.

- Good storage area- all teas must be stored in an air-tight, light-proof container in order for the tea to be fresh with every brew. Placing it in a cool dry place are also the best conditions for tea.
- Share the tea- when I saw the amazing results tea had on my body I couldn't wait to share it with friends and family so I recommend you give it a try. Enjoying a fresh cup of tea with friends and family gives you great pleasure and helps you appreciate the little things in life a lot more.
- Using the right teapot- While seemingly irrelevant at first, the material of the teapot being used also affects the quality of the infusion. Materials like iron or Chinese yixing ware are superb at retaining heat over long periods of time which is best when preparing black tea. Green and white teas, on the other hand need a vessel that stays cooler, such as porcelain.

Tea Cleanse Diet Plan

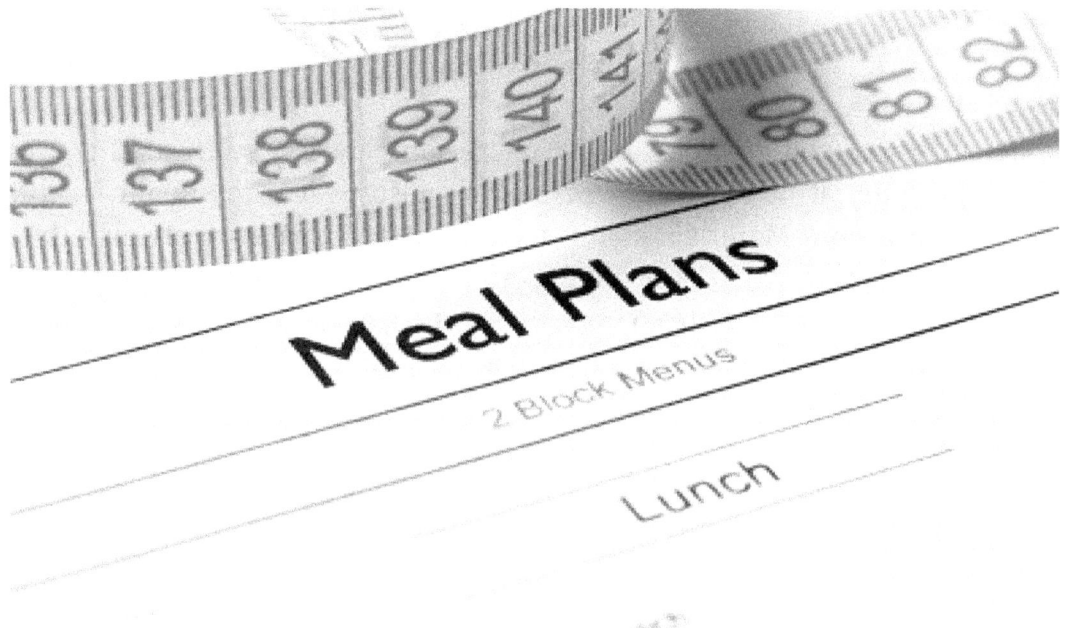

The word "diet" is often associated with several different stigmatisms. Diets are associated with a desire to lose weight, deprivation of your favorite foods, or achieving an unrealistically thin body type of low fat percentage. However, this definition is often misleading. These three things do not encompass the full meaning of the word diet. A diet, according to the definition in this book, is choosing foods for health and nutrition. This will help your body instead of harming it and help you achieve great results without you starving or being deprived from your favorite foods. This book is about this kind of diet- a healthful one. It is not about consuming a ridiculously low amount of calories or trying to obtain a smaller body type. Instead, this book is about making healthy choices in your diet, whether you are trying to lose a few pounds or just looking to achieve total wellness through your diet a tea cleanse diet plan can and will help you reach your desired goals. Here is what you will get from this diet.

Improving Mental and Emotional Health

In the last decade, several studies have been done that link the foods we eat to our mental and emotional health. Among this was a study that compared Western diets against diets of meats and vegetables in other countries. The study found that those eating a Western diet that is typically filled with processed and red meats, takeout foods, sugary snacks, and pre-packaged meals are linked to a higher occurrence of mental health problems such as bipolar disorder, depression, and anxiety. It also was linked to a higher level of stress. Eliminating these harmful foods from your diet is a must and it will improve mental/emotional health significantly. You will fill more at peace, healthier, more able to take on each day and focused throughout your many activities.

Lowering the Risk of Disease and Improving Weight Loss

When you eat a healthier diet that includes various teas and full of nutritional foods it is also linked to a lower occurrence of disease. This includes a lower risk of obesity-related diseases such as cardiovascular problems and diabetes, as well as a lower risk of everything from asthma to eczema. The reason that our diet is believed to affect the occurrence of so many different diseases is because our traditional Western diets do not nurture the trillion microorganisms that live in our body. Many of these organisms live in the stomach and digestive tract and a tea cleanse is one of the best ways to improve that. They are responsible for keeping our body healthy- by balancing out the bad bacteria and keeping us healthy. Unfortunately, the diets that most Americans consume cause the diversity of the good bacteria to be significantly lowered. Our diet can also raise the occurrence of bad bacteria and throw off the balance of the internal ecosystem that lives in our stomach. While it is not the only cause of the following diseases, it has been shown to cause asthma, allergies, restless leg syndrome, fibromyalgia, acne, and other diseases in some people.

The bottom line is that our diets can affect nearly every aspect of our well-being. From our physical health to our mental health, the foods we eat do make a difference and that's why when on this tea cleanse it's extremely important to complement your tea beverages with healthy foods. In this chapter, we will discuss a healthy diet- one that is directed at improving your physical, mental, and emotional health so that you have a better quality of life and what's great about this is that doing just that will have you melting away pounds in as little as one week with no exercise.

Day 1 Meal Plan

Breakfast

1 cup green tea
1 medium apple
1 Scramble egg burrito

Morning Snack (Brunch)

1 cup cantaloupe

Lunch

Asian salad with crispy chicken

Afternoon Snack

1 cup blackberries
1 cup oolong tea

Dinner

1 plate Confetti pesto pasta

Post Dinner

Pepper mint tea

Day 1 Recipes

Scramble Egg Burrito

Ingredients (Prepares 2 rolls)

- 2 large eggs, or equivalent egg substitute
- 1 tablespoon 1% low-fat milk
- 1 teaspoon chopped fresh cilantro
- 1/8 teaspoon kosher salt
- Dash of coarsely ground black pepper
- Cooking spray
- 1/2 teaspoon butter
- 4 tablespoons reduced-fat shredded cheddar cheese, divided
- 2 (8-inch) fat-free flour tortillas, heated
- 4 tablespoons chopped seeded tomato, divided
- 2 tablespoons bottled chunky salsa, divided

Preparation Instructions

STEP 1: place the first five ingredients (egg, milk, cilantro, salt, pepper) in a bowl and whisk them.

STEP 2: get your nonstick skillet and coat it with cooking spray. Add in some butter and let melt over a medium heat. When the butter has melted pour your egg mixture into the skillet and stir with a spatula to scramble.

STEP 3: sprinkle 2 tablespoons cheese down the center of one tortilla; add half of the scrambled egg, 2 tablespoons tomato, and 1 tablespoon chunky salsa.

STEP 4: wrap it all together burrito-style.

More info- breakfast is the best way there is to get ready for a good day and this scramble egg burrito is just what you need to give you a boost of energy with 15 grams of protein and less than 260 calories per burrito.

And if you want to cut back on cholesterol and fat the egg white can be used instead of the whole egg. Fat-free milk and fat-free cheese are also good ways to further cut back on fat.

Asian Salad with Crispy Chicken

Ingredients

- 2 chicken breast fillets, skinless, cut into 1" cubes
- 1 tablespoon canola oil
- 1 tablespoon sesame oil
- 3 cups shredded Savoy (curly) Cabbage, optional Napa Cabbage
- 2 cups chopped Romaine lettuce
- 1 carrot, peeled, sliced
- 2 tablespoons sesame seeds, lightly toasted

Dressing:

- 2 tablespoon honey
- 2 teaspoons Dijon mustard
- 1 tablespoon lite soy sauce, low sodium, optional Bragg's Liquid Aminos
- 1 tablespoon rice wine vinegar
- 1 tablespoon freshly squeezed lemon juice

Preparation Instructions

STEP 1: place a dry nonstick skillet over a medium fire and place sesame seeds in for about 5 minutes or until fragrant.

STEP 2: In a medium skillet add canola and sesame oil, the chicken cubes will be cooked here on a medium-high heat for about 10 minutes or until cooked through and crispy.

STEP 3: place the cooked chicken, lettuce, cabbage, and carrots in a bowl and sprinkle over with sesame seeds.

STEP 4: mix all the dressing ingredients together and whisk until they all are properly combined.

STEP 5: spread the dressing over the salad and mix and toss to combine.

More info- complementing this tea cleanse diet is an Asian salad with crispy chicken. Not only is this meal delicious but also is less than 200 calories per serving (1 cup) and fills you with the protein, fiber and other nutrients that you need to continue with your activities for the day.

Confetti Pesto Pasta

Ingredients (serves 4)

- 4 cups whole grain linguine
- 1 1/2 cup green beans
- 1 pint cherry tomatoes, halved
- 1 1/2 cup diced chicken breast
- 1/4 cup pesto sauce
- 1/4 tsp each salt and pepper
- 1/4 cup shredded Parmesan cheese

Preparation Instructions

STEP 1: combine 1 pint cherry tomatoes, 1 1/2 cups cooked green beans, 1 1/2 cups diced chicken breast, 1/4 cup pesto sauce, and 1/4 tsp each salt and pepper.

STEP 2: add 4 cups cooked linguine.

STEP 3: garnish with 1/4 cup shredded Parmesan and serve.

More Info- if you're craving pasta then this meal is just what you need to settle your cravings without adding to much fat or calories to your diet. This delicious meal serves 4 so the entire family can enjoy. One serving of confetti pesto pasta will fill up your hunger and offer you plenty of protein to keep you feeling full. Not only is the nutritional value of this meal amazing but it's only at 395 calories and can be prepared within 30 minutes.

Day 2 Meal Plan

Breakfast

1 cup green tea
2 banana corn muffins
1 cup skim milk
1 medium orange

Morning Snack (Brunch)

1 fruit and nut granola bar

Lunch

Strawberry, avocado salad with strawberry balsamic dressing
1 cup almond milk

Afternoon Snack

6 Ounces Nonfat Vanilla or Lemon Yogurt, Sweetened with Low-Calorie
Sweetener

Dinner

1 plate Garlic turkey-broccoli stir-fry
½ cup blackberries

Post Dinner

White tea

Day 2 Recipes

Banana Corn Muffins

Ingredients

- 1/2 cup mashed ripe banana
- 1/2 cup 2% reduced-fat milk
- 1 (8 1/2-ounce) package corn muffin mix (such as Jiffy)
- Cooking spray

Preparation Instructions

STEP 1: start by preheating your oven to 350 degrees

STEP 2: add the banana, milk and muffin mix in a bowl and stir until moist.

STEP3: coat 6 muffin cups with cooking spray and spoon the batter evenly into it.

STEP 4: place in oven for 22 minutes (or until a wooden pick is inserted and comes out clean) at a heat of 350 degrees.

STEP 5: let cool after it's removed from the oven and enjoy.

More Info- these banana corn muffins are a sweet treat that can go with almost anything. This reduced milk in this recipe can also be substituted with fat-free milk which has 5 grams less fat. With calories of only 199 per muffin you can't go wrong with this sweet treat.

Strawberry, avocado salad with strawberry balsamic dressing

Ingredients (serves 2)

Salad:
- 4 cups fresh baby spinach leaves
- 4 cups arugula
- 1/2 cup strawberries, sliced
- 1/3 cup avocado, sliced
- 1/3 cup blueberries or blackberries

Dressing:
- 1/2 cup strawberries (roughly cut)
- 1 tbsp. balsamic vinegar
- 1 dash stevia (optional)

Preparation Instructions

STEP 1: add all the dressing ingredients into a food processor or blender and process until it's well blended.

STEP 2: grab a bowl and add all salad ingredients in.

STEP 3: toss with dressing and serve

More Info- top with strawberries for a more aesthetic appeal. This meal is definitely a nutritional lunch that is tasty. With very little calories (135 per serving) the strawberry, avocado salad with strawberry balsamic dressing makes weight loss easy and delightful.

Garlic turkey-Broccoli Stir-Fry

Ingredients (serves 4)

- 2 teaspoons sesame oil, divided
- 1 (1-pound) turkey tenderloin, cut into thin strips
- 1 cup fat-free, less-sodium chicken broth
- 4 garlic cloves, minced
- 1 1/2 tablespoons cornstarch
- 1/4 teaspoon crushed red pepper
- 1/4 teaspoon salt
- 1 red bell pepper, cut into thin strips
- 2 cups fresh broccoli florets
- 1 (8-ounce) can sliced water chestnuts, drained
- 2 tablespoons low-sodium soy sauce

Preparation Instructions

STEP 1: on a medium-high heat, place a nonstick skillet and add 1 tablespoon of sesame oil when it's hot (ensure the pan is coated evenly with the oil).

STEP 2: add the turkey and stir-fry until the turkey is no longer pink in the center, about 5 minutes. Then remove from the skillet and set aside.

STEP 3: in a bowl combine the broth with the next 4 ingredients (garlic cloves, cornstarch, and red pepper, salt) and stir until the cornstarch has dissolved then set aside.

STEP 4: add the remainder of the sesame oil to the pan followed by adding the broccoli and red bell pepper strips. Stir-fry this for 1 minute and add water chestnuts; stir-fry for 30 another seconds.

STEP 5: raise the heat to high. Stir the broth mix and add to the pan with turkey, soy sauce and any accumulated juices.

STEP 6: bring to a boil and let cook until it has slightly thickened for about 1-2 minutes.

STEP 7: let cool and enjoy!

More Info- the garlic turkey-broccoli stir-fry is an easy to cook meal that will stimulate your taste buds and give you a great deal of nutrients. With 27.5 grams of protein and 262 calories this is an amazing complementary meal to your tea cleanse that will help you shed pounds without having you starving. Share this with the family or friends and they too will be surprised something so tasty can be so good for your health.

Day 3 Meal Plan

Breakfast

1 cup oolong tea
1 cup skim milk
1 cup Cheerios cereal
1 medium apple

Morning Snack (Brunch)

1 medium orange

Lunch

BBQ chicken cob salad

Afternoon Snack

1 cup grapes
Green tea

Dinner

1 bowl quinoa with black beans
1 cup skim milk
1 medium nectarine

Post Dinner

1 cup peppermint tea
½ cup blackberries

Day 3 Recipes

BBQ Chicken Cob Salad

Ingredients (serves 1)

- 3 ounces boneless, skinless chicken breast
- 2 tablespoons barbecue sauce (divided)
- 2 slices turkey bacon (chopped)
- 1 ½ cups chopped romaine lettuce
- 1 hardboiled egg white (chopped)
- ¼ cup chopped grape tomatoes
- ¼ avocado (chopped)

Preparation Instructions

STEP 1: begin by preheating the oven to 350 degrees.

STEP 2: brush the chicken with 1 tablespoon of barbecue sauce and place it in a baking dish that has been sprayed with nonstick spray.

STEP 3: bake the chicken until the there is no pink color, about 25 minutes.

STEP 4: cook the bacon according to the package directions.

STEP 5: place the romaine on a plate and add the other cooked ingredients. Drizzle with the other tablespoon of barbecue sauce and enjoy.

More Info- with only 280 calories this is one meal you wouldn't want to share. This delightful protein packed lunch will keep you feel great and full all throughout the afternoon until dinner.

Quinoa with Black Beans

Ingredients (serves 4)

- 1 tablespoon olive oil
- 1 medium sweet or yellow onion, diced
- 2 cloves garlic, minced
- 3/4 cup quinoa (uncooked), rinsed (red or white will work)
- 1 (15 ounce) can black beans(low sodium preferred), drained and rinsed
- 1 teaspoon chili powder
- 1 teaspoon cumin
- 1/4 teaspoon crushed red pepper flakes (more or less to taste)
- 1/2 teaspoon black pepper
- Kosher or sea salt to taste
- 1 (4.5 ounce) can diced green chilis
- 1 (10 ounce) can diced tomatoes
- 1/2 cup freshly chopped cilantro
- 1 3/4 cup vegetable broth, low sodium

Preparation Instructions

STEP 1: place a large skillet on a medium-low heat and add in 1 tablespoon of olive oil. Sauté the diced onions in the olive oil until they are tender, about 4 minutes.

STEP 2: add garlic and sauté once more for an addition minute. Follow this by adding the remaining ingredients in the order from the list above.

STEP 3: cover, bring to a boil and adjust the heat to a low boil and cook until the all the liquid has been absorbed, about 15-20 minutes.

STEP 4: remove from the heat and let cool for 5 minutes with the cover on before serving.

STEP 5: uncover and fluff the quinoa with a spoon then serve.

More Info- the combination of the different ingredients in this dish makes it a favorite for Mexican food lovers. This meal is a vegetarian, gluten free bowl of joy with super-foods quinoa and black beans which contains vitamins and minerals that improve health across the board. Holding only 4 grams of fat and 200 calories per serving (1 cup) how can this delicious dish not be included as a favorite?

Day 4 Meal Plan

Breakfast

1 cup green tea
1 bowl Oatmeal with apples, hazelnuts and flaxseeds
1 cup almond milk
½ grapefruit

Morning Snack (Brunch)

1 fruit and nut granola bar

Lunch

1 bowl super-food salad
1 cup honeydew melon

Afternoon Snack

1 cup blackberries
1 cup skim milk

Dinner

1 bowl slow cooker chicken noodle soup
½ almonds

Post Dinner

White tea

Day 4 Recipes

Oatmeal with Apples, Hazelnuts and Flaxseed

Ingredients (serves 6)

- 1/4 cup hazelnuts
- 3 cups fat-free milk
- 1 1/2 cups regular oats
- 1 1/2 cups diced Granny Smith apple (about 1 medium)
- 1/3 cup ground flaxseed
- 1/2 teaspoon ground cinnamon
- 1/4 teaspoon salt
- 1/2 teaspoon vanilla extract
- 3 tablespoons brown sugar
- 3 tablespoons slivered almonds

Preparation Instructions

STEP 1: start by pre-heating the oven to 350 degrees

STEP 2: bake hazelnuts on a baking sheet for 15 minutes at 350 degrees, stirring once.

STEP 3: place the nuts on a towel and roll it up in order to rub off the skins. Then chop the nuts and set them aside.

STEP 4: mix the milk and the next 5 ingredients (oats, diced apple, flaxseed, cinnamon and salt) in a saucepan.

STEP 5: bring the mixture to a boil over a medium heat and add it vanilla and stir. Cover, reduce the heat and simmer until it's thick, about 5 minutes.

STEP 6: sprinkle with hazelnuts, almonds and brown sugar. Let cool and enjoy!

More Info- if you get hazelnuts where the skins are already off you can just go straight to chopping them and skip the steps prior to that. This breakfast is a great meal to start the day and get the energy, nutrients and taste bud stimulation you know you want and need. This breakfast has less than 260 calories per serving (2/3 cup) and almost 10 grams of protein so trust me when I say you're doing your body a favor when you eat this.

Super-Food Salad

Ingredients (serves 6)

- One head of kale
- 1/4 cup pine nuts
- 1/2 cup dried cranberries or currants
- Juice of 1 lemon
- 1/4 cup extra-virgin olive oil
- Pinch of kosher or sea salt

Preparation Instructions

STEP 1: remove the large stems of the kale leaves and discard.
STEP 2: chop the kale leaves and add to a large bowl also adding pine nuts, dried cranberries or currants.

STEP 3: add the lemon juice to the bowl, sprinkle it with salt and drizzle with olive oil. Toss to combine and serve.

More Info- kale is a super-food and there are an abundance of reasons why this vegetable is so great. Based on information from Web MD, one cup of kale provides 5 grams of fiber, 15% of calcium and B6, 40% magnesium, 180% vitamin A, 200% vitamin C and 1,020 % vitamin k with only 36 calories. This beneficial veggie is a no-brainer when improving health. Did I mention that it's also contains antioxidants such as beta-carotene and folic acid. The salad itself contains 162 calories and taste great when garnished with parmesan cheese if you want to mix it up.

Beef and Broccoli Stir-Fry

Ingredients (serves 4)

- 1 pound pre-cut beef for stir-fry
- 2 garlic cloves, smashed
- 1 tablespoon minced fresh ginger
- 2 tablespoons soy sauce
- 1 bunch broccoli (about 1 lb.)
- 2 tablespoons vegetable oil
- 1/2 cup water
- 1 1/2 cups beef broth
- 2 tablespoons cornstarch
- 1 cup fresh mung bean sprouts

Preparation Instructions

STEP 1: add together in a bowl beef, garlic, soy sauce and ginger and let stand.

STEP 2: rinse the broccoli and cut into florets. Then trim and peel the stems and cut into ¼ inch thick slices.

STEP 3: in a large nonstick skillet heat 1 tablespoon of oil on a high heat. When the skillet is hot add in the broccoli, stems and florets and stir-fry for 2 minutes.

STEP 4: add ½ cup of water to the pan and stir until the water evaporates then transfer the broccoli to the plate.

STEP 5: add the remainder of the oil to the pan followed by the beef and stir-fry for 3 minutes.

STEP 6: stir together the cornstarch and the broth. Add the mixture to the meat and stir-fry for another 3 minutes or until the sauce has thickened.

STEP 7: add broccoli and bean sprouts, then cook, stirring, until heated through for about 2 minutes.

More Info- for this recipe to get the most favor out of your dish you should use fresh vegetables when cooking. This Asian meal only contains 266 calories per serving and is a great source of vitamins with 32 grams.

Day 5 Meal Plan

Breakfast

1 cup oolong tea
1 breakfast taco
1 cup skim milk
1 medium orange

Morning Snack (Brunch)

6 Ounces Nonfat Vanilla or Lemon Yogurt, Sweetened with Low-Calorie Sweetener

Lunch

1 bowl creamy pesto pasta salad
1 cup grapes
1 cup skim milk

Afternoon Snack

1 cup cantaloupe
1 cup green tea

Dinner

1 plate salmon and arugula salad
1 cup strawberries

Post Dinner

1 cup peppermint tea

Day 5 Recipes

Quick Breakfast Taco

Ingredients (serves 2)

- 2 corn tortillas
- 1 tablespoon salsa
- 2 tablespoons shredded reduced-fat Cheddar cheese
- 1/2 cup liquid egg substitute, such as Egg Beaters

Preparation Instructions

STEP 1: spread cheese and salsa over the tortilla and heat in the microwave or oven until the cheese has melted, about 30 seconds.

SREP 2: place a nonstick skillet (coated with cooking spray) over a medium heat. Add the egg to the skillet and cook, stirring until the eggs has been cooked through, about 90 seconds.

STEP 3: divide the egg between the tacos and serve.

More Info- this satisfying and healthy breakfast option has only 239 calories and as you may have observed is protein packed which will keep you full until your net meal.

Creamy Pesto Pasta Salad

Ingredients

- 1 (12 ounce box) whole wheat Rotini pasta, optional penne or ziti
- 1 cup low-fat Greek yogurt, plain (I used 2% which is reflected in the nutritional data)
- 1/2 cup Pesto
- 3/4 cups (coarsely chopped) sun-dried tomatoes, packed in olive oil and drained

Preparation Instructions

STEP 1: cook the pasta according to the package directions. Drain the pasta and rinse with cold water and leave to chill.

STEP 2: mix the yogurt with the pesto and add it to the pasta. Toss the mixture so it can be evenly coated.

STEP 3: add sun-dried tomatoes and toss again. Place in the fridge until ready to serve.

More Info- It's recommended that to serve this pasta salad immediately or soon after preparing because the olive oil, in the pesto, tends to get thick after several hours in the fridge. Also when cutting the sun-dried tomatoes, the ends that tend to be tough can be discarded. The creamy pesto pasta salad has only 190 calories per serving and is a delicious meal.

Salmon and Arugula Salad

Ingredients

- ¼ (each) kosher salt and black pepper
- 1 tablespoon olive oil
- 2 bunches arugula
- 1 (15.5) ounce can chickpeas, rinsed
- ¼ small red onion, sliced
- ½ cucumber, sliced
- ¼ cup kalamata olives, sliced
- ¼ cup vinaigrette
- ¾ pound skinless salmon fillet

Preparation Instructions

STEP 1: begin by seasoning the salmon with the black pepper and kosher salt.

STEP 2: add the olive oil to a nonstick skillet over a medium-high heat.

STEP 3: cook the salmon until opaque throughout, about 5 minutes per side then let cool and flake.

STEP 4: toss in the rest of the ingredients (arugula, chickpeas, onion, cucumber, olives and vinaigrette) and serve.

More Info- the salmon and arugula salad is a healthy, delicious low calorie meal you can enjoy that will have you super satisfied at the end of the day.

Now, we have come to the end of your diet plan. The meal plan of days 1-5 will be repeated for days 6-10 in the same order completing your 10 day journey. Continuing with the tea cleanse every few weeks or so will create a better and healthier life for you. If all you're looking for is to shed a few pounds before an event or activity then do just that, but if you're looking for that paradigm shift continue with the cleanse until you're comfortable and have developed your-self to the "you" that you want.

Conclusion

Thank you again for downloading this book!

I hope this book was able to help you to understand how to lose weight, build muscle and improve your health with carb cycling. The wealth of information presented will prove to be of great value once the steps have been followed. Choose a cycle, create your workout routine, get motivated and TAKE ACTION. No more excuses, no more postponements, and no more bullshitting your-self saying you can't do it because you can. This is your life and it's up to you to make the change so make the change. Implementing the ideas in this book will place in your hand the mold that is needed to shape your-self in any way you want. Keep focus and do your best because your best is a lot better than you think it is.

Finally, if you enjoyed this book, then I'd like to ask you for a favor, would you be kind enough to leave a review for this book on Amazon? It'd be greatly appreciated!

Thank you and good luck. Wishing you massive success!

What Else is There?

Just as there are many methods to find an answer in mathematics there are also other ways of achieving weight loss success with different methods. It's true that there is a lot of fake stuff out there offering amazing results but it is also true that there are a few authentic and genuine means of losing weight. One that I know which have worked wonders in the lives of many is carb cycling. My friend Peter David has done a great job helping people sculpt their bodies into a masterpiece, well at least what they consider to be a master piece. After all it's about what you want....right? Although it's difficult to get a hold of David (yes I refer to him by his surname) you can get his newly published book *"Carb Cycling: The Revolutionary Weight Loss Plan Designed to Shed Pounds."* Personally I love learning new ways to tackle problems and not having the body you want is a problem so if you're looking for another way to tackle problems you have with health and weight loss get the book. I was able to get a copy before it was published (thanks David) so I can tell you that there are solid techniques in there to help you out. Here's a preview:

Preview Of *"Carb Cycling: The Revolutionary Weight Loss Plan Designed to Shed Pounds"*

Chapter 1: Carb Cycling Overview

Over the years carb cycling has gained popularity after slipping under the radar. This mainstream diet strategy provides many benefits especially for people looking for fat loss and muscle growth. So the question is what is carb cycling? In its basic format carb cycling is the alteration of foods containing carbohydrates in order to effectively reduce fat gain and boost your metabolism. What does this mean, you ask?

Carbohydrates have been accused for many years of being the evil entity behind obesity and weight gain in general, but how true is that ideology? If you really understand the purposes carbohydrates serves and know a few techniques to deal with them (which will be explained thoroughly in this book) then you will see just as clearly as I do how simple it is to consume carbs and have them working for you rather than against you.

The carb cycling plans/strategies are based on low carb days, no carb days and high carb days. The alteration between the levels of carbohydrates in your diet at just the right times is what causes your body to respond differently to the consumption of carbohydrates. But let's talk about what the days involve while going through the carb cycling process.

Low carb diets and high carb diets have been used and tested to see what benefits they have in health and weight loss but carb cycling is a result of the merge that took place between these two diets in order to maximize benefits and reduce any negative effects. Although both low carb and high carb diets have their advantages, long term use of these diets can bring about negative results on your health. Combining these two diets eliminates majority of those risky side effects and provides significant assistance in health and weight loss.

While coming up with the right plan to achieve your goals carb cycling alters specific things in your diet but there are certain things with carb cycling which stay the same no matter what carb cycling strategy you go with. On a daily basis here are the basics:

- Each day contains exactly 5 meals
- Within 30 minutes of waking up you should have a high carb breakfast. Your breakfast should include a substantial amount of carbs (1.5 cups for women and 2 cups for men), protein (3 ounces for women and 5 ounces for men) and non-starchy veggies (2 cups for women and 3 cups for men).
- Depending on the carb cycling plan you're following your day will include the recommended amount of carbs to consume for each meal as well as the approved foods for the day.
- Your meals throughout the day must be eaten at intervals of 3 hours of each other.
- Each day of your carb cycling plan you must drink plenty of water (approximately 1 gallon)

Why does Carb Cycling Work?

As we have discussed carb cycling is a shift from different levels of carbohydrates over a period of time and the foods which are consumed in this diet obviously plays an important role in reducing weight, building muscle and making you feel healthy. The foods and meals have been specifically chosen because of the benefits of the combination of protein, carbohydrates and healthy fats they provide. It may seem strange that carbohydrates, proteins and fats actually help with weight loss but they do with the right combination and when taken at the right time. Let me explain why:

To find out more about "Carb Cycling: The Revolutionary Weight Loss Plan Designed to Shed Pounds" by Peter David go to: **http://bit.ly/carb-cycling-plan**